NATURAL AND HEALTHY

HAIR GROWTH

a holistic guide to growing healthy and beautiful hairs with herbs

Dr Philip Ortner

Table of Contents

CHAPTER 1

Introduction

Healthy hair is more than just a cosmetic feature; it's a reflection of our overall well-being. Think about it – when your hair looks good, you feel good. It's a boost to your confidence, a sign of vitality, and an expression of your personality. In this chapter, we'll dive into the importance of having healthy hair, touch upon some common hair issues that many people face, and introduce the wonderful world of herbal remedies that can transform the health and appearance of your mane.

Overview of the Significance of Healthy Hair

Let's begin by understanding why healthy hair matters so much. Your hair is not just dead cells growing out of your scalp; it's a dynamic part of your body that undergoes constant renewal. Beyond aesthetics, healthy hair is an indicator of your internal health. Just like your skin or nails, your hair reflects what's happening inside your body.

When your body is in good shape, it shows in your hair. Nutrient-rich blood nourishes the hair follicles, promoting growth and strength. On the flip side, poor nutrition, stress, and various health issues can negatively impact your hair. Ever notice how your hair might lose its luster or become more prone to breakage during times of stress or illness? That's your body signaling that something might be amiss.

Beyond health, hair is deeply tied to cultural and personal identity. Different hairstyles can convey a sense of style, tradition, or rebellion. Hair can be a canvas for self-expression, whether it's through a bold color choice, a funky cut, or simply letting it flow naturally.

Brief Explanation of Common Hair Issues

Now that we understand the significance of healthy hair, let's acknowledge that not everyone wakes up with a perfect mane every day. Hair issues are incredibly common, and most people have experienced at least one of them at some point.

Hair loss is a major concern for many individuals. Whether it's due to genetics, hormonal changes, or lifestyle factors, losing hair can be distressing. It's not just about vanity – for many, it's a source of insecurity and can affect self-esteem.

On the other end of the spectrum, some struggle with hair that seems impossible to control. Frizz, split ends, and dryness can turn a good hair day into a bad one in no time. Environmental factors like sun exposure, pollution, and harsh styling practices contribute to these issues.

Dandruff and itchy scalp are also common culprits. These issues can be both embarrassing and uncomfortable, leading to a constant battle with different shampoos and treatments.

Understanding these common hair issues is crucial because it sets the stage for exploring solutions. It's not just about covering up the problems but addressing the root causes for long-term solutions.

Introduction to the Benefits of Herbal Remedies

This is where herbal remedies come into play. Imagine a world where you can address your hair issues without relying on harsh chemicals or expensive salon treatments. Herbs, with their natural properties, have been used for centuries across various cultures to promote hair health.

Herbal remedies offer a holistic approach to hair care. Instead of just focusing on external symptoms, they work from the inside out, nourishing your scalp and hair follicles. This not only addresses existing issues but also prevents future problems.

One significant advantage of herbal remedies is their gentleness. Unlike some commercial products that can strip your hair of its natural oils, herbal solutions often work in harmony with your body. They can soothe irritated scalps, provide essential nutrients, and promote a healthy environment for hair growth.

Herbs come in various forms – from oils and masks to teas and tinctures. This versatility allows you to choose the method that best fits your lifestyle and preferences. Whether you're a fan of DIY projects or prefer ready-made herbal products, there's a herbal solution for everyone.

Moreover, herbal remedies often have a lower environmental impact compared to mass-produced, chemical-laden hair care products. By opting for natural solutions, you contribute to a healthier planet while taking care of your hair.

In the upcoming chapters, we'll explore specific herbs known for their hair benefits, learn how to create herbal hair care products, and integrate these remedies into a personalized hair care routine. It's time to unlock the secrets of herbal wisdom for vibrant, healthy hair. Get ready to embark on a journey that goes beyond just aesthetics – it's about nurturing your hair and embracing the beauty of natural solutions.

CHAPTER 2

Understanding Hair Growth

Anatomy of the Hair Follicle

Let's start by unraveling the mystery of hair growth, beginning with the tiny powerhouse called the hair follicle. Imagine the hair follicle as a miniature factory beneath your skin, responsible for producing each strand of hair. These follicles are scattered all over your scalp and are even present in other parts of your body, albeit producing finer and shorter hair.

The hair follicle is like a bulb planted in the skin. At its base is the papilla, a small, nourishing blood vessel that supplies nutrients to the growing hair. Picture the papilla as the roots of a plant, soaking up essential nutrients from the soil to fuel growth. As the cells in the papilla divide, they create the hair strand we see on the surface.

Now, surrounding the papilla is the hair matrix, a region where the cells rapidly divide, pushing the older cells upward. As these cells move up, they undergo a process of keratinization, essentially transforming into the protein keratin, which is the primary component of your hair. By the time these cells reach the surface of the skin, they have become the visible hair we all know.

The sebaceous gland, a tiny oil-producing factory attached to the follicle, plays a crucial role as well. It secretes sebum, an oil that moisturizes and protects the hair. When everything works harmoniously, you get a healthy, shiny mane.

Hair Growth Cycles

Understanding hair growth involves recognizing that your hair is not in a perpetual state of growth. Instead, it undergoes cycles, much like the changing seasons. There are three main phases in the hair growth cycle:

1. **Anagen Phase (Growth Phase):** This is the active phase where your hair is busy growing. During this

period, the cells in the hair matrix divide rapidly, pushing the hair strand upward. The length of the anagen phase varies from person to person, but on average, it lasts between two to seven years. The longer this phase, the longer your hair can potentially grow.

2. **Catagen Phase (Transition Phase):** Think of this as a brief pit stop in the growth journey. The catagen phase lasts only a few weeks and marks the transition between the active growth phase and the resting phase. During this time, the hair follicle shrinks, and the hair detaches from the blood supply. It's a natural pause before the next cycle begins.

3. **Telogen Phase (Resting Phase):** Now, your hair takes a break. In this phase, which lasts around three months, the hair is no longer growing, but it's still attached to the follicle. About 10-15% of your hair is in this phase at any given time. Eventually, the hair strand falls out, and the follicle gears up

for a new cycle with the growth of a new hair strand.

Understanding these cycles helps explain why you might not see drastic changes in your hair length every day. Some hairs are actively growing, while others are in a resting phase. This cycling process ensures a continuous supply of new hair.

Factors Affecting Hair Growth

Now that we've explored the intricacies of the hair follicle and growth cycles, it's time to consider the numerous factors that influence this complex process. Hair growth isn't solely determined by your genes; it's a delicate dance between genetics, lifestyle, and environmental factors.

1. **Genetics:** Your genetic code plays a significant role in determining the length, thickness, and growth patterns of your hair. If your parents or grandparents had a particular hair type, there's a

good chance you might share similar characteristics.

2. **Hormones:** Hormones, those chemical messengers that regulate various bodily functions, also have a say in your hair's fate. Androgens, a group of hormones that includes testosterone, can influence hair growth. For instance, dihydrotestosterone (DHT), a derivative of testosterone, can shrink hair follicles and lead to hair loss, especially in genetically predisposed individuals.

3. **Nutrition:** Remember that papilla we talked about earlier, the one responsible for nourishing the growing hair? Well, it needs the right nutrients to do its job effectively. A well-balanced diet rich in vitamins, minerals, and proteins provides the building blocks for healthy hair. Deficiencies in essential nutrients can hinder the hair growth process.

4. **Stress:** Yes, stress can affect your hair. Chronic stress may push more hair into the resting phase, leading to increased shedding. Additionally, stress

can contribute to hormonal imbalances that impact hair health.

5. **Age:** As much as we'd like to defy the aging process, it does influence our hair. Hair growth tends to slow down as we age, and the diameter of individual hair strands may decrease, leading to thinner-looking hair.

6. **Health Conditions:** Certain health conditions, such as thyroid disorders, autoimmune diseases, and polycystic ovary syndrome (PCOS), can affect hair growth. Medications used to treat these conditions may also have an impact.

7. **Environmental Factors:** Exposure to harsh environmental conditions, pollution, and excessive sunlight can take a toll on your hair. It's not just your skin that needs protection – your hair can benefit from some TLC too.

Understanding these factors empowers you to make informed choices about your hair care routine. Whether you're adjusting your diet, managing stress, or choosing the right products, you have the tools to promote a healthy hair environment.

In the subsequent chapters, we'll delve into the exciting world of herbal remedies and how they can address some of these factors naturally. By combining this knowledge with practical tips, you'll be well-equipped to embark on a journey toward healthier, more vibrant hair. Get ready to nurture those follicles and let your hair thrive!

CHAPTER 3

Common Causes of Hair Loss

Overview of Common Reasons for Hair Loss

Hair loss is a universal concern that can affect people of all ages and genders. While it's entirely normal to shed some hair daily (in fact, we lose around 50 to 100 hairs each day), excessive hair loss can be distressing. In this chapter, we'll explore the common reasons behind hair loss and delve into the role that environmental factors, lifestyle choices, genetic influences, stress, and hormonal changes play in this intricate process.

Firstly, it's crucial to understand that hair loss is a symptom rather than a condition on its own. It can be a result of various underlying factors, and identifying the root cause is essential for effective treatment and prevention.

Common reasons for hair loss include

1. **Androgenetic Alopecia (Genetic Hair Loss):**
   Also known as male-pattern baldness or female-pattern baldness, this is the most common cause of hair loss. It's hereditary and can affect both men and women. In men, it often presents as a receding hairline and bald spots, while women may experience overall thinning.

2. **Telogen Effluvium:** This is a condition where more hair than usual enters the resting (telogen) phase of the hair growth cycle. It often occurs after a significant physical or emotional stressor, such as surgery, illness, or childbirth. The good news is that this type of hair loss is usually temporary.

3. **Alopecia Areata:** An autoimmune condition where the immune system mistakenly attacks hair follicles, leading to hair loss. This can result in small, round patches of baldness on the scalp or other areas of the body.

4. **Traction Alopecia:** Caused by tight hairstyles that pull on the hair, such as ponytails, braids, or cornrows. Over time, this constant pulling can damage the hair follicles and lead to hair loss.

5. **Medical Conditions:** Certain medical conditions and treatments, such as thyroid disorders, lupus, and chemotherapy, can contribute to hair loss. It's essential to address the underlying health issue to improve hair health.

6. **Nutritional Deficiencies:** Lack of essential nutrients, particularly iron, zinc, and vitamins A and D, can impact hair growth. A well-balanced diet is crucial for maintaining healthy hair.

Now, let's delve into the environmental factors, lifestyle choices, genetic influences, stress, and hormonal changes that can contribute to these common causes of hair loss.

Environmental Factors, Lifestyle, and Genetic Influences

1. **Environmental Factors:** Your hair, just like your skin, can be affected by the environment. Exposure to pollution, harsh weather conditions, and ultraviolet (UV) radiation can damage your hair. Pollutants in the air can build up on your scalp and hair, potentially leading to inflammation and hair loss.

   Protecting your hair from these environmental stressors can involve simple measures such as wearing a hat on sunny days, using a scarf in harsh weather, and washing your hair regularly to remove accumulated pollutants.

2. **Lifestyle Choices:** Your daily habits can significantly impact the health of your hair. Over-styling, excessive use of heat tools, and aggressive brushing can lead to physical damage, weakening the hair shaft and making it more prone to breakage.

Additionally, poor lifestyle choices like a lack of exercise, inadequate sleep, and smoking can contribute to hair loss. Regular exercise promotes good blood circulation, including to the scalp, which is essential for delivering nutrients to the hair follicles.

Quitting smoking is not only beneficial for your overall health but can also improve the condition of your hair. Smoking restricts blood flow, which can negatively affect the health of your hair follicles.

3. **Genetic Influences:** The genes you inherit from your parents play a significant role in determining your susceptibility to hair loss. If your family has a history of androgenetic alopecia or other hereditary conditions, you may be more prone to experiencing hair loss.

While you can't change your genetic makeup, understanding your family history can help you be proactive in managing and preventing hair loss. Early intervention and adopting healthy habits can slow down or mitigate the impact of genetic factors on your hair.

The Impact of Stress and Hormonal Changes on Hair Health

1. **Stress:** We've all heard the phrase "pulling your hair out in frustration," and there's a reason for that – stress can indeed contribute to hair loss. High-stress levels can push more hair follicles into the resting phase, leading to increased shedding.

   Chronic stress can also contribute to conditions like trichotillomania, where individuals compulsively pull out their hair. This behavioral aspect of stress can further exacerbate hair loss.

   Managing stress is crucial for maintaining overall health, and it can have positive effects on your hair as well. Practices such as meditation, deep breathing exercises, and engaging in hobbies can help alleviate stress and promote a healthier head of hair.

2. **Hormonal Changes:** Hormones play a crucial role in regulating various bodily functions, including hair growth. Fluctuations in hormone levels, especially androgens, can impact the hair growth cycle.

For example, during pregnancy, women experience a surge in hormones that can lead to thicker, more luscious hair. However, after childbirth, when hormone levels drop, some women may experience postpartum hair loss. This type of hair loss is typically temporary, and the hair usually regrows within a few months.

Hormonal changes can also occur during menopause, affecting the thickness and texture of hair. Hormone replacement therapy (HRT) is sometimes used to manage these changes and their impact on hair.

Understanding the interplay of these factors gives you the knowledge to make informed choices about your lifestyle and habits, promoting healthier hair. In the subsequent chapters, we'll explore the benefits of herbal remedies in addressing these common causes of hair loss. By incorporating natural solutions into your routine, you can nurture your hair and promote a vibrant, resilient mane. Get ready to embrace the power of herbs on your journey to healthier, more beautiful hair.

CHAPTER 4

Power of Herbs in Hair Care

Introduction to the History of Herbal Remedies for Hair Growth

Imagine a time long before the colorful bottles of commercial hair products lined the shelves. Our ancestors, in tune with nature, turned to the abundance of plants around them to care for their hair. This chapter is a journey into the historical roots of herbal remedies for hair growth, exploring how civilizations across the globe recognized the power of herbs in nurturing and beautifying their locks.

The use of herbs for hair care is deeply woven into the fabric of human history. Ancient cultures, from the Egyptians to the Greeks and Ayurvedic practitioners in India, recognized the therapeutic properties of various plants for maintaining healthy hair. Herbs were not only used for cosmetic purposes but also for their medicinal value in addressing specific hair and scalp concerns.

In Egypt, for instance, historical records indicate that both men and women used a variety of herbal concoctions to enhance the health and aesthetics of their hair. Olive oil, castor oil, and aloe vera were among the favored ingredients for promoting hair growth and preventing hair loss.

In Ayurveda, the traditional system of medicine in India, herbs like Amla (Indian Gooseberry), Brahmi, and Neem have been integral to hair care for centuries. These herbs were believed to balance the doshas (energies) in the body, promoting overall well-being, including the health of the hair and scalp.

Fast forward to the present day, and the resurgence of interest in natural and holistic approaches to health and beauty has brought herbal remedies back into the spotlight. As we explore the benefits of herbs for hair care, it's important to recognize that this wisdom has been passed down through generations, a testament to the enduring efficacy of herbal treatments.

Explanation of How Herbs Nourish and Strengthen Hair

So, what is it about herbs that makes them potent allies in the quest for healthy, luscious hair? To understand this, let's break down how herbs work to nourish and strengthen the hair from root to tip.

1. **Scalp Nourishment:** The health of your hair starts at the roots – the scalp. Herbs like Aloe Vera, known for its soothing properties, can moisturize the scalp, reducing dryness and itchiness. This creates a conducive environment for hair growth by supporting the health of hair follicles.

2. **Improved Blood Circulation:** Many herbs, when applied topically or ingested, have the ability to enhance blood circulation. Improved blood flow to the scalp means better delivery of oxygen and

nutrients to the hair follicles. This, in turn, promotes hair growth and strengthens the roots.

3. **Balancing Oil Production:** An imbalance in the production of sebum (natural scalp oil) can lead to oily or dry scalp conditions. Herbs like Rosemary and Lavender are known for their ability to regulate sebum production, helping maintain a healthy scalp environment.

4. **Reducing Inflammation:** Inflammation of the scalp can contribute to hair loss. Herbs such as Chamomile and Calendula have anti-inflammatory properties that can soothe the scalp and reduce inflammation, creating an environment conducive to hair growth.

5. **Fortifying Hair Strands:** Herbs are rich in vitamins, minerals, and antioxidants that can fortify the hair shaft. For example, Nettle Leaf is packed with iron and other essential nutrients that contribute to stronger, healthier hair.

6. **Moisture Retention:** Proper hydration is crucial for hair health. Herbs like Hibiscus and

Marshmallow Root have emollient properties that help retain moisture in the hair, preventing dryness and breakage.

7. **Cleansing and Detoxification:** Just as we detoxify our bodies, our hair can benefit from a detox too. Herbs like Bentonite Clay and Shikakai have cleansing properties that can remove build-up from the scalp and hair, promoting a clean and healthy environment.

Overview of Key Nutrients Found in Herbs

Now, let's explore the treasure trove of nutrients that herbs offer for hair health. These natural wonders provide a holistic approach to nourishing your hair, delivering a combination of vitamins, minerals, and other beneficial compounds.

1. **Vitamins:**

   o **Vitamin A:** Found in herbs like Aloe Vera, it promotes a healthy scalp and supports the production of sebum.

- **Vitamin C:** Abundant in herbs like Amla, it aids in collagen production, vital for maintaining the structure of hair.
- **Vitamin E:** Present in herbs like Rosemary, it acts as an antioxidant, protecting hair from damage.

2. **Minerals:**

- **Iron:** Herbs like Nettle Leaf are rich in iron, essential for preventing hair loss and promoting growth.
- **Zinc:** Found in herbs like Pumpkin Seed, it helps maintain the health of hair follicles.
- **Silica:** Horsetail Herb is a source of silica, a mineral that contributes to hair strength and elasticity.

3. **Fatty Acids:**

- **Omega-3 Fatty Acids:** Flaxseed and Chia Seeds, often used in herbal hair remedies, provide omega-3 fatty acids that support scalp health and hair shine.

4. **Antioxidants:**

- **Flavonoids:** Herbs like Green Tea are rich in flavonoids, which have antioxidant properties that protect hair from free radical damage.

- **Polyphenols:** Present in herbs like Sage, polyphenols contribute to overall hair health and vitality.

5. **Proteins:**

- **Keratin-Boosting Herbs:** Bamboo Extract is a natural source of silica, which aids in the production of keratin, the protein that forms the structure of the hair.

Understanding the specific nutrients in herbs allows you to choose remedies tailored to your hair's needs. Whether you're looking to strengthen, moisturize, or stimulate growth, there's an herbal solution waiting to nourish your hair naturally.

CHAPTER 5

Top Herbs for Hair Growth

Embarking on a journey into herbal hair care is like stepping into a lush garden of nature's remedies. In this chapter, we'll explore the detailed profiles of key herbs renowned for their hair growth benefits. Each herb has its unique properties, offering a bouquet of nourishment and care for your precious locks. We'll unravel the benefits these herbs bring to your hair health and guide you on how to incorporate them into your routine through oils, masks, and teas.

Aloe Vera

Profile: Aloe vera, often referred to as the "plant of immortality," is a succulent plant known for its gel-filled leaves. The gel, when extracted, is a transparent, cooling substance with a myriad of benefits.

Benefits for Hair Health:

- **Soothing and Moisturizing:** Aloe vera's hydrating properties make it an excellent choice for soothing a dry and itchy scalp. It helps lock in moisture, preventing dryness that can lead to dandruff and hair breakage.

- **Balancing pH Levels:** Aloe vera helps maintain the natural pH balance of the scalp, creating an environment conducive to hair growth.

- **Strengthening Hair Strands:** Rich in vitamins and minerals, aloe vera nourishes the hair shaft, adding strength and luster to your locks.

How to Use:

- **Aloe Vera Gel:** Apply the gel directly to your scalp and hair, leaving it on for about 30 minutes before washing it off with a mild shampoo.

- **Aloe Vera Hair Mask:** Mix aloe vera gel with other nourishing ingredients like coconut oil or honey to create a hydrating hair mask.

Hibiscus:

Profile: Hibiscus, with its vibrant and trumpet-shaped flowers, is not just a garden beauty but a treasure trove for hair care. Both the flowers and leaves of the hibiscus plant are used for their hair-loving properties.

Benefits for Hair Health:

- **Stimulating Hair Growth:** Hibiscus is rich in vitamins A and C, promoting the production of collagen necessary for hair growth.
- **Preventing Hair Fall:** The amino acids in hibiscus strengthen hair roots, reducing hair fall and making your strands more resilient.
- **Natural Conditioner:** Hibiscus acts as a natural conditioner, leaving your hair soft and manageable.

How to Use:

- **Hibiscus Oil:** Infuse hibiscus flowers in a carrier oil like coconut or olive oil, creating a nourishing oil blend.

- **Hibiscus Hair Mask:** Blend hibiscus petals with yogurt or aloe vera gel to create a hair mask that moisturizes and revitalizes your hair.

Ginseng:

Profile: Ginseng, an herb native to Asia, has been a staple in traditional medicine for centuries. Known for its adaptogenic properties, ginseng helps the body adapt to stress and brings a multitude of benefits to hair care.

Benefits for Hair Health:

- **Improved Blood Circulation:** Ginseng stimulates blood flow to the scalp, providing more oxygen and nutrients to hair follicles.
- **Preventing Hair Loss:** The active compounds in ginseng help reduce hair loss and promote hair regrowth.
- **Balancing Oil Production:** Ginseng helps regulate sebum production, preventing an overly oily or dry scalp.

How to Use:

- **Ginseng Infused Oil:** Infuse dried ginseng roots in a carrier oil to create a potent oil that can be massaged into the scalp.
- **Ginseng Tea Rinse:** Brew ginseng tea and use it as a hair rinse after shampooing to invigorate the scalp.

Rosemary:

Profile: Rosemary, with its fragrant needle-like leaves, is a culinary herb that also works wonders for hair health. Its essential oil and extracts have been used for centuries in traditional medicine.

Benefits for Hair Health:

- **Stimulating Hair Growth:** Rosemary is known to increase blood circulation to the scalp, promoting hair growth.
- **Preventing Dandruff:** Its antimicrobial properties help in preventing dandruff and maintaining a healthy scalp.

- **Strengthening Hair:** Rosemary strengthens hair strands, reducing breakage and split ends.

How to Use:

- **Rosemary Oil:** Infuse rosemary leaves in a carrier oil or use rosemary essential oil to massage the scalp.
- **Rosemary Hair Rinse:** Boil rosemary leaves in water, let it cool, and use it as a final hair rinse after washing.

Nettle Leaf:

Profile: Nettle leaf, often considered a pesky weed, is a powerhouse of nutrients when it comes to hair care. Rich in vitamins and minerals, nettle leaf has been used traditionally to address various health concerns, including hair issues.

Benefits for Hair Health:

- **Promoting Hair Growth:** Nettle leaf is loaded with iron, promoting healthy hair growth and preventing hair loss.
- **Strengthening Hair:** Its high mineral content, including silica, strengthens hair strands and adds shine.
- **Reducing Dandruff:** Nettle leaf has anti-inflammatory properties that can help soothe and reduce dandruff.

How to Use:

- **Nettle Leaf Tea:** Prepare nettle leaf tea and use it as a hair rinse or incorporate it into your herbal hair care routine.
- **Nettle Leaf Infused Oil:** Infuse nettle leaves in a carrier oil to create a nourishing oil for the scalp and hair.

How to Use These Herbs in Various Forms (Oils, Masks, Teas)

1. **Herbal Oils:**
   - *Infusion Method:* Infuse herbs like hibiscus, rosemary, or nettle leaf in a carrier oil (coconut, olive, jojoba) for several weeks. Strain the herbs, and you're left with a potent herbal oil that can be massaged into the scalp.
   - *Essential Oils:* Add a few drops of essential oils like rosemary or ginseng to your regular carrier oil for a boost of herbal goodness.

2. **Herbal Hair Masks:**
   - *Fresh Herb Masks:* Blend fresh herbs like aloe vera, hibiscus, or ginseng with yogurt or aloe vera gel to create nourishing masks. Apply to damp hair and leave for 30 minutes before washing.
   - *Dry Herb Masks:* Powder dried herbs like nettle leaf or ginseng and mix with water or

aloe vera gel to create a paste. Apply as a mask for a revitalizing treatment.

3. **Herbal Teas and Rinses:**

   - *Teas for Drinking:* Brew herbal teas like nettle leaf or ginseng for consumption. The internal benefits of these teas can contribute to overall hair health.

   - *Teas for Rinsing:* Prepare herbal teas and use them as a final hair rinse after shampooing. Allow the tea to cool before pouring it over your hair.

Incorporating these herbs into your hair care routine allows you to tap into the bountiful offerings of nature. Experiment with different combinations and formulations to find what works best for your hair type and specific needs. The beauty of herbal remedies lies in their versatility and the ability to tailor them to your unique hair journey. Get ready to infuse your locks with the goodness of these top herbs, nurturing them from root to tip for vibrant, healthy hair.

CHAPTER 6

Creating Herbal Hair Care Products

Welcome to the hands-on chapter of your herbal hair care journey! In this section, we'll delve into the world of DIY (Do It Yourself) herbal hair care products, exploring simple yet effective recipes for herbal hair masks, oils, and rinses. We'll also discuss essential tips for selecting and preparing herbs, ensuring you get the most out of nature's bounty while maintaining safe and effective application practices.

DIY Recipes for Herbal Hair Masks, Oils, and Rinses

1. **Herbal Hair Masks:**
   - *Aloe Vera and Hibiscus Mask:*
     - Ingredients: Aloe vera gel, hibiscus petals (fresh or dried), yogurt.

- Method: Blend a handful of hibiscus
      petals with aloe vera gel and yogurt.
      Apply the mixture to damp hair,
      focusing on the scalp and ends. Leave
      for 30 minutes before washing with a
      mild shampoo.
  - *Nettle Leaf and Rosemary Strengthening Mask:*
    - Ingredients: Nettle leaf powder,
      rosemary essential oil, honey.
    - Method: Mix nettle leaf powder with
      a few drops of rosemary essential oil
      and honey to create a thick paste.
      Apply to hair and leave for 30-45
      minutes before washing.

2. **Herbal Hair Oils:**
   - *Ginseng-Infused Oil:*
     - Ingredients: Dried ginseng roots,
       carrier oil (coconut, olive).
     - Method: Infuse dried ginseng roots in
       a carrier oil for several weeks. Strain

the oil and massage it into the scalp. Leave it on for at least an hour or overnight before washing.

- o *Rosemary and Lavender Hair Oil:*
  - Ingredients: Rosemary leaves, lavender essential oil, jojoba oil.
  - Method: Infuse fresh rosemary leaves in jojoba oil. Add a few drops of lavender essential oil. Apply to the scalp and hair, leave for at least 30 minutes, and wash as usual.

3. **Herbal Hair Rinses:**

- o *Chamomile and Calendula Soothing Rinse:*
  - Ingredients: Chamomile flowers, calendula petals.
  - Method: Steep chamomile flowers and calendula petals in hot water to create a tea. After shampooing, pour the tea over your hair as a final rinse.
- o *Green Tea and Aloe Vera Clarifying Rinse:*

- Ingredients: Green tea leaves, aloe vera gel.
- Method: Brew green tea, let it cool, and mix with aloe vera gel. Use it as a hair rinse after washing to clarify and soothe the scalp.

Tips for Selecting and Preparing Herbs:

1. **Choose Quality Herbs:**
   - Opt for organic or wildcrafted herbs whenever possible to ensure they are free from pesticides and chemicals.
   - Fresh herbs can be a great choice, but dried herbs are often more convenient and have a longer shelf life.

2. **Consider Your Hair Type and Needs:**
   - Different herbs cater to various hair concerns. For example, if you have dry hair, you might choose herbs like aloe vera or hibiscus for their moisturizing properties. If you're aiming for increased circulation,

herbs like rosemary or ginseng could be beneficial.

3. **Mix and Match:**

   - Don't be afraid to experiment with different herb combinations to find what works best for your hair. Combining herbs can create a synergy of benefits.

4. **Be Mindful of Sensitivities:**

   - Perform a patch test before using any new herb to ensure you don't have an allergic reaction.

   - If you have known sensitivities or allergies, research each herb carefully to avoid potential adverse effects.

5. **Use Quality Carrier Oils:**

   - When infusing herbs in oils, choose high-quality carrier oils like coconut, olive, jojoba, or sweet almond oil.

   - Cold-pressed and unrefined oils retain more of their natural properties.

6. **Store Herbs Properly:**

- o Keep dried herbs in a cool, dark place to maintain their potency.
- o Store infused oils in dark glass bottles to prevent degradation from light.

Guidelines for Safe and Effective Application:

1. **Patch Testing:**
   - o Before applying any new herbal product to your scalp or hair, perform a patch test on a small area of skin to check for adverse reactions.

2. **Consistency is Key:**
   - o Herbal remedies often require consistent use to see results. Incorporate them into your hair care routine regularly for the best outcome.

3. **Avoid Overuse:**
   - o While herbs are generally safe, using them excessively may lead to product build-up or

potential sensitivities. Follow recommended guidelines and listen to your hair's needs.

4. **Balance DIY with Commercial Products:**

   o Herbal DIY products can be fantastic additions to your routine, but don't hesitate to complement them with commercial products if needed. A balanced approach ensures comprehensive care.

5. **Be Patient:**

   o Herbal remedies work gradually, and it may take some time to notice significant changes. Patience is key when transitioning to a more natural hair care routine.

6. **Rinse Thoroughly:**

   o When using herbal masks or oils, make sure to rinse your hair thoroughly to remove any residue. This prevents build-up and ensures your hair stays clean and healthy.

Embarking on the journey of creating your herbal hair care products is an exciting and empowering step toward natural, holistic hair care. With these DIY recipes, tips for herb selection, and application guidelines, you have the tools to customize your hair care routine according to your unique needs and preferences. Enjoy the process of nurturing your hair with the goodness of herbs, and let your locks flourish in their newfound natural vitality.

CHAPTER 7

Incorporating Herbs into Your Hair Care Routine

Congratulations on reaching the pinnacle of your herbal hair care journey! In this chapter, we'll guide you through building a personalized herbal hair care regimen, offering tips for maintaining a healthy scalp, and exploring how to seamlessly combine herbs with conventional hair care products. It's time to make herbal care an integral part of your routine, creating a nourishing and holistic approach to beautiful, vibrant hair.

Building a Personalized Herbal Hair Care Regimen:

1. **Identify Your Hair Needs:**
    - Assess your hair type, whether it's dry, oily, or a combination, and identify any specific

concerns like dandruff, hair loss, or lack of shine.

o Consider your hair goals – whether you want to promote growth, strengthen strands, or simply maintain overall health.

2. **Select Herbs Tailored to Your Goals:**

o Choose herbs that align with your specific hair needs. For example, if you're focusing on growth, herbs like aloe vera, ginseng, and rosemary can be beneficial. For moisturizing, hibiscus and aloe vera are excellent choices.

3. **Incorporate a Variety of Herbs:**

o Create a diverse herbal repertoire. Rotate different herbs in your routine to provide a range of nutrients and benefits to your hair.

o Experiment with combinations to find what works best for you. For instance, you might combine a strengthening herb like nettle leaf with a soothing herb like chamomile for a balanced approach.

4. **Establish a Routine:**

   o Integrate herbal care into your existing hair care routine. Whether it's a weekly mask, a monthly oil treatment, or a daily herbal rinse, consistency is key to seeing results.

5. **Listen to Your Hair:**

   o Pay attention to how your hair responds to different herbs. If you notice positive changes or, conversely, any adverse effects, adjust your routine accordingly.

   o Adapt your herbal regimen based on seasonal changes and shifts in your hair's condition.

Tips for Maintaining a Healthy Scalp:

1. **Gentle Scalp Massage:**

   o Incorporate regular scalp massages into your routine using your fingers or a soft brush. This helps stimulate blood flow, promoting a healthy scalp environment.

2. **Proper Cleansing:**

- Keep your scalp clean by washing your hair regularly. Choose a gentle, sulfate-free shampoo to avoid stripping natural oils.
- Consider alternating between herbal hair rinses and commercial shampoos to balance cleansing with natural nourishment.

3. **Balanced Moisture:**

- Maintain a balanced moisture level in your hair and scalp. If you have a dry scalp, herbs like aloe vera and hibiscus can provide hydration. For an oily scalp, herbs with astringent properties like rosemary and sage can help regulate oil production.

4. **Avoid Excessive Heat Styling:**

- Limit the use of heat styling tools as excessive heat can contribute to scalp dryness and hair damage. If you must use heat, apply a protective herbal serum or oil beforehand.

5. **Protect Your Hair:**

- Shield your hair from harsh environmental conditions. Cover your hair in extreme weather, use a swim cap in chlorinated water, and protect your hair from the sun to prevent damage.

6. **Hydrate and Nourish from Within:**

- Stay hydrated and maintain a balanced diet rich in vitamins and minerals to support overall hair health. Consider herbal teas or supplements containing herbs like nettle leaf or horsetail for an internal boost.

Combining Herbs with Conventional Hair Care Products:

1. **Choose Compatible Products:**

- Select commercial products that complement your herbal routine. For example, if you're using an herbal oil, choose a sulfate-free shampoo that won't strip away the natural oils.

2. **Customize Your Routine:**

- o Tailor your routine to incorporate both herbal and conventional products. You might use an herbal hair rinse after shampooing with a commercial product or apply an herbal mask before using your regular conditioner.

3. **Gradual Transition:**

- o If you're transitioning from conventional to herbal products, consider a gradual shift. Start by incorporating one herbal product at a time and observe how your hair responds.

4. **Balance as Needed:**

- o Balance is key when combining herbal and conventional products. Too much of one may counteract the benefits of the other. Pay attention to your hair's needs and adjust your routine accordingly.

5. **Be Mindful of Ingredients:**

- o Check the ingredients in your commercial products to avoid conflicts with herbs. Some ingredients, like silicones, may create a barrier that prevents herbal benefits from reaching your hair.

6. **Experiment with Blending:**

   o Get creative by blending herbal concoctions with your favorite store-bought products. For instance, add a few drops of rosemary essential oil to your regular conditioner for an herbal boost.

Incorporating herbs into your hair care routine is a delightful and empowering experience. As you build a personalized regimen, remember that the journey is as important as the destination. Listen to your hair, embrace the versatility of herbs, and enjoy the transformative process of nurturing your locks with nature's gifts.

With this comprehensive guide, you're equipped to embark on a holistic herbal hair care journey. From DIY recipes and tips for selecting herbs to building a personalized regimen and blending with conventional products, you have the tools to cultivate a vibrant, healthy mane. Embrace the rhythm of nature and your unique hair needs, and watch as your herbal-infused routine unveils the beauty within each strand.

CHAPTER 8

Lifestyle Tips for Healthy Hair

Welcome to the final chapter of your holistic hair care journey! In this section, we'll explore the crucial role of lifestyle factors in promoting healthy hair. From the foods you eat to the way you manage stress, these aspects play a significant role in the vitality and resilience of your locks. Let's dive into the key lifestyle tips for maintaining a healthy mane.

The Role of Nutrition and Hydration in Promoting Hair Growth

Imagine your hair as a garden, and your body as the soil – what you feed it directly influences the health of what grows. The same principle applies to your hair. Here's a breakdown of how nutrition and hydration impact your locks:

1. **Protein for Stronger Strands:**

    o   Hair is primarily made up of a protein called keratin. Incorporating protein-rich foods into your diet, such as lean meats, fish, eggs, and plant-based sources like beans and lentils, provides the building blocks for stronger, more resilient hair.

2. **Iron for Preventing Hair Loss:**

    o   Iron deficiency is a common cause of hair loss. Include iron-rich foods like spinach, lentils, red meat, and fortified cereals in your diet to ensure your body has an adequate supply of this essential nutrient.

3. **Omega-3 Fatty Acids for Shine:**

    o   Omega-3 fatty acids found in fatty fish, flaxseeds, chia seeds, and walnuts contribute to the health and shine of your hair. They nourish the scalp and hair follicles, promoting a vibrant mane.

4. **Vitamins and Antioxidants for Overall Health:**

o Vitamins A, C, and E, along with antioxidants, play a crucial role in maintaining overall health, including that of your hair. Incorporate a variety of colorful fruits and vegetables, such as carrots, berries, and leafy greens, into your diet.

5. **Hydration for Moisture:**

   o Just as your skin needs hydration, so does your hair. Drinking an adequate amount of water ensures that your hair stays moisturized from the inside out. Dehydration can lead to dry and brittle hair.

Exercise and Its Impact on Hair Health

Physical activity doesn't just benefit your body; it's a boon for your hair as well. Here's how staying active contributes to a healthy mane:

1. **Improved Blood Circulation:**

   o Exercise gets your blood pumping, and this increased circulation benefits your scalp.

Improved blood flow means more oxygen and nutrients are delivered to your hair follicles, promoting growth and overall health.

2. **Stress Reduction:**

   o Regular exercise is a potent stress buster. Stress is a known factor in hair loss, and finding ways to manage it can contribute to maintaining a fuller head of hair.

3. **Balanced Hormones:**

   o Hormonal imbalances can impact hair health. Exercise helps regulate hormone levels, including those that affect the hair growth cycle.

4. **Sweat and Detoxification:**

   o Sweating during exercise helps unclog hair follicles and promotes detoxification. Just be sure to wash your hair afterward to remove any accumulated sweat and prevent potential scalp issues.

5. **Yoga for Mind-Body Harmony:**

o Practices like yoga not only provide physical exercise but also incorporate stress-relieving techniques. Certain yoga poses can stimulate the scalp and contribute to healthier hair.

Stress Management Techniques for Maintaining a Healthy Mane

Stress is a silent saboteur of hair health. Chronic stress can lead to conditions like telogen effluvium, where hair follicles shift prematurely into the resting phase, resulting in increased hair shedding. Here are stress management techniques to keep your mane stress-free:

1. **Meditation and Mindfulness:**
   o Taking a few minutes each day to practice meditation or mindfulness can significantly reduce stress levels. Focus on your breath, be present in the moment, and let go of tension.

2. **Deep Breathing Exercises:**

o Deep, slow breathing activates the body's relaxation response. Practice deep breathing exercises to calm your nervous system and reduce stress.

3. **Regular Exercise:**

    o As mentioned earlier, physical activity is a powerful stress reducer. Find a form of exercise you enjoy, whether it's jogging, dancing, or yoga, and make it a regular part of your routine.

4. **Quality Sleep:**

    o Lack of sleep can contribute to stress and impact your overall well-being, including the health of your hair. Prioritize getting enough quality sleep each night.

5. **Creative Outlets:**

    o Engaging in creative activities, whether it's painting, writing, or playing a musical instrument, can be therapeutic and provide an outlet for stress.

6. **Social Support:**

- o Share your thoughts and concerns with friends, family, or a support network. Having a strong social support system can alleviate stress and contribute to better mental health.

7. **Aromatherapy:**

    - o Certain scents, like lavender and chamomile, are known for their calming effects. Incorporate aromatherapy into your routine through essential oils or scented candles to create a soothing environment.

8. **Time Management:**

    - o Organize your tasks and prioritize what needs to be done. Effective time management can help reduce feelings of overwhelm and stress.

Incorporating these lifestyle tips into your daily routine creates a holistic approach to hair care. As you nourish your body with the right nutrients, stay active, and manage stress, your hair will reflect the health and vitality of your overall well-being. Remember, the journey to healthy hair is not just about external treatments but also about embracing a lifestyle that supports your body and mind. Enjoy the process, and revel in the beautiful, healthy mane that is the result of your mindful and holistic care.

CONCLUSION

Embracing Herbal Wisdom for Vibrant Locks

As we conclude this journey into the realm of herbal wisdom for vibrant locks, it's time to reflect on the key herbal remedies and the profound benefits they offer to nurture and beautify your hair. From the soothing embrace of aloe vera to the strengthening powers of nettle leaf, the holistic approach to herbal hair care has opened a door to a world where nature's gifts harmonize with the needs of your precious mane.

Recap of Key Herbal Remedies and Their Benefits

1. **Aloe Vera:** The cooling balm for a dry scalp and a natural hydrator, aloe vera fosters an environment where your hair can thrive, combining moisture and strength.

2. **Hibiscus:** With its vibrant petals, hibiscus emerges as a stimulating force, promoting hair growth,

preventing hair fall, and offering a natural conditioner for luscious locks.

3. **Ginseng:** Hailing from ancient traditions, ginseng steps forward with its ability to improve blood circulation, prevent hair loss, and balance oil production for a healthier scalp.

4. **Rosemary:** The fragrant herb that invigorates, rosemary stimulates hair growth, prevents dandruff, and strengthens strands, leaving you with a crown of resilient and radiant locks.

5. **Nettle Leaf:** Once dismissed as a weed, nettle leaf takes center stage, providing essential nutrients for promoting growth, strengthening hair, and reducing dandruff.

As we've explored, the power of herbs lies not only in their individual attributes but in their synergy. Blending these herbs in oils, masks, and rinses allows you to tailor your hair care routine, addressing specific needs and delighting in the diverse benefits nature has to offer.

Encouragement to Embrace a Holistic Approach to Hair Care

Beyond the concoctions and applications, herbal hair care invites us to embrace a holistic approach, recognizing that the health of our hair is intricately connected to our overall well-being. It's a dance between the external nourishment we provide through herbal remedies and the internal care we cultivate through lifestyle choices.

Nourishing your hair from the inside out involves mindful nutrition, ensuring your body receives the essential building blocks for strong and vibrant locks. It means staying hydrated, acknowledging that the moisture your hair craves begins with the water you drink.

Physical activity becomes not just a routine but a celebration of vitality, as exercise stimulates blood flow, balances hormones, and contributes to the overall health of your scalp and hair.

Stress management transforms from a necessity into an art, with practices like meditation, deep breathing, and creative outlets serving as tools to maintain a serene and stress-free environment for your hair to flourish.

Closing Thoughts on the Journey to Healthy, Beautiful Hair

As you tread the path towards healthy, beautiful hair, remember that this journey is a celebration of self-care. It's a process of discovering what works best for you, listening to the needs of your hair, and finding joy in the rituals of herbal wisdom.

In the quest for vibrant locks, patience becomes your ally. Herbal remedies work gradually, weaving their magic over time. Allow your hair to unfold its natural beauty, trusting in the potency of the herbs and the care you invest.

In closing, let your hair be a reflection of the love and attention you've showered upon it. Each strand tells a story of the herbal treasures it has embraced, the nourishment it has received, and the holistic care that has become a daily ritual.

May your journey to healthy, beautiful hair be a source of empowerment and self-discovery. Embrace the wisdom of herbs, honor the uniqueness of your locks, and revel in the beauty that unfolds when nature and care intertwine. Your vibrant locks are not just a testament to external radiance but a reflection of the inner harmony you've cultivated on this enriching journey into herbal wisdom. Cheers to the beauty that blossoms when you embrace the holistic magic of herbal hair care!